POCKET ATLAS OF NORMAL CT ANATOMY OF THE HEAD AND BRAIN

Pocket Atlas of Normal CT Anatomy of the Head and Brain

Anton N. Hasso, M.D.

Director of Neuroradiology
Loma Linda University School of Medicine
Loma Linda, California

Miyuki Shakudo, M.D.

Fellow, Department of Radiology
Osaka City University Medical School
Osaka, Japan

Raven Press **New York**

Raven Press, 1185 Avenue of the Americas, New York, New York 10036

Made in the United States of America

Library of Congress Cataloging-in-Publication Data

Hasso, Anton N.
    Pocket atlas of normal CT anatomy of the head and brain / Anton N.
    Hasso.
        p.   cm.
    Includes bibliographical references.
    ISBN 0-88167-663-2
    1. Brain—Tomography—Atlases.   2. Head—Tomography—Atlases.
I. Title.
    [DNLM: 1. Brain—anatomy & histology—atlases.   2. Brain—radi-
ography—atlases.   3. Head—anatomy & histology—atlases.   4.
Head—radiography—atlases.   5. Tomography, X-Ray Computed—atlases.   WE 17 H3555p]
QM455.H337   1990
611'.81'0222—dc20
DNLM/DLC   90-8707
for Library of Congress   CIP

The material contained in this volume was submitted as previously unpublished material, except in the instances in which credit has been given to the source from which some of the illustrative material was derived.

Great care has been taken to maintain the accuracy of the information contained in the volume. However, neither Raven Press nor the editors can be held responsible for errors or for any consequences arising from the use of the information contained herein.

9 8 7 6 5 4 3 2 1

Preface

Computed tomography (CT) has evolved into a mature technology that has widespread applications throughout the human body. Prior to CT, complex motion tomography was particularly useful for the evaluation of the temporal bone and skull base. The remaining structures of the head and brain were less optimally visualized. With the advent of high-resolution CT, all the remarkable anatomic details of the head and brain are routinely imaged. The soft tissue and bony structures are equally well seen with the utilization of appropriate "window settings" and algorithms.

The images were obtained with commercial CT scanners during routine clinical studies. The labeling was referenced according to several standard atlases and textbooks including: Correlative Sectional Anatomy of the Head and Neck, by Joseph R. Thompson and Anton N. Hasso, The C.V. Mosby Company, St. Louis, 1980; Radiology: Diagnosis, Imaging and Intervention, edited by Juan M. Taveras and Joseph T. Ferrucci, J.B. Lippincott Company, Philadelphia, 1987; and Modern Neuroradiology (Volume 3), Computed Tomography of the Head and Neck, edited by Thomas H. Newton, Anton N. Hasso, and William P. Dillon, Raven Press, New York, 1988.

This atlas is intended to portray all the normal

anatomy that is incorporated into routine CT images of the head and brain. In addition to detailing the central nervous system structures in adults and children, there are illustrations of the skull base, temporal bone, and sella. The value of CT image reconstruction is exemplified in a sagittal series of temporal bone anatomy.

This book will be of interest to radiologists, neurologists, neurosurgeons, and otolaryngologists.

Acknowledgments

The authors are grateful to the CT technologists at Loma Linda University Medical Center for the dedication and efforts to produce consistent quality scans. We also acknowledge that assistance of Mr. James Simmons in reproduction of the publication prints and Mrs. Penny Thomas in manuscript preparation.

Contents

Brain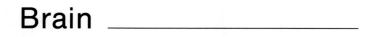

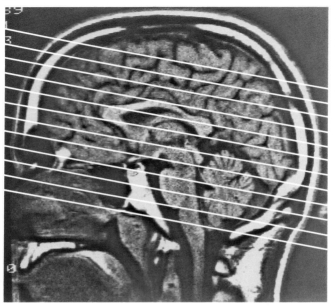

FIG. 1.
EMI plane.

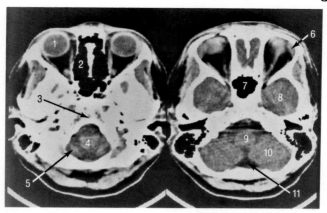

FIG. 2.
1, ocular bulb
2, ethmoid sinus
3, clivus
4, medulla
5, cerebellar tonsil
6, lacrimal gland
7, sphenoid sinus
8, temporal lobe
9, medulla
10, cerebellar hemisphere
11, cisterna magna

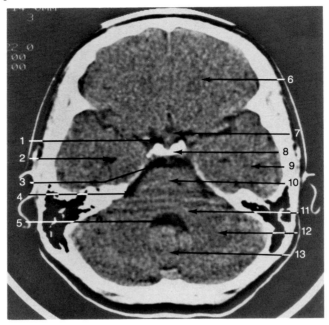

FIG. 3.
1, suprasellar cistern
2, temporal horn
3, prepontine cistern
4, cerebellopontine angle cistern
5, 4th ventricle
6, frontal lobe
7, optic chiasm
8, dorsum sellae
9, temporal lobe
10, pons
11, middle cerebellar peduncle
12, cerebellar hemisphere
13, cerebellar vermis

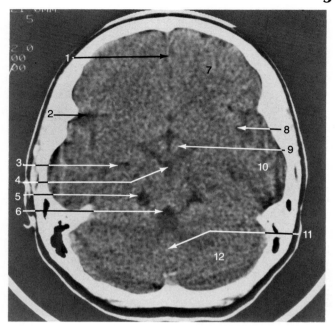

FIG. 4.
1, interhemispheric fissure
2, Sylvian fissure
3, temporal horn
4, interpeduncular cistern
5, ambient cistern
6, 4th ventricle (upper portion)
7, frontal lobe
8, insula
9, hypothalamus
10, temporal lobe
11, cerebellar vermis
12, cerebellar hemisphere

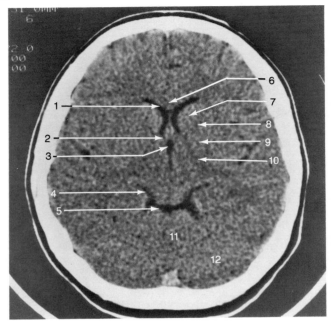

FIG. 5.
1, frontal horn
2, foramen of Monro
3, 3rd ventricle
4, ambient cistern
5, quadrigeminal cistern
6, genu of corpus callosum
7, head of caudate nucleus
8, anterior limb of internal capsule
9, lentiform nucleus
10, posterior limb of internal capsule
11, cerebellar vermis
12, cerebellar hemisphere

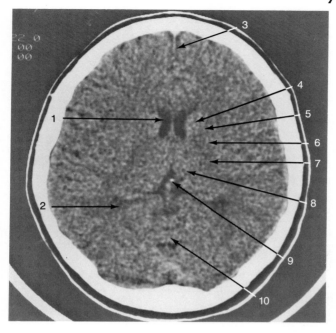

FIG. 6.
1, frontal horn
2, temporal horn
3, falx
4, head of caudate nucleus
5, anterior limb of internal capsule
6, lentiform nucleus
7, posterior limb of internal capsule
8, thalamus
9, pineal gland
10, cerebellar vermis

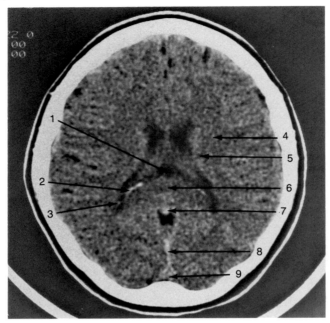

FIG. 7.
1, cavum vergae
2, choroid plexus
3, trigone
4, corona radiata
5, body of caudate nucleus
6, corpus callosum
7, vein of Galen
8, falx
9, superior sagittal sinus

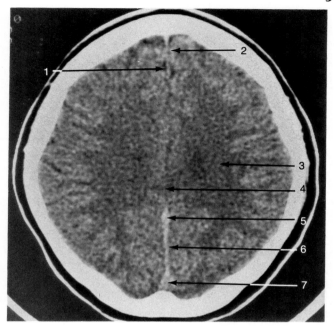

FIG. 8.
1, interhemispheric fissure
2, falx
3, centrum semiovale
4, corpus callosum
5, inferior sagittal sinus
6, falx
7, superior sagittal sinus

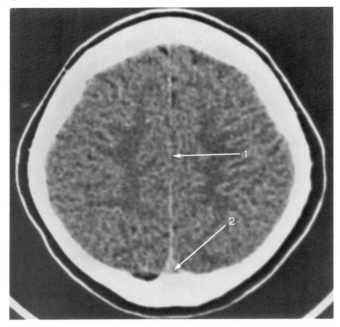

FIG. 9.
1, falx
2, superior sagittal sinus

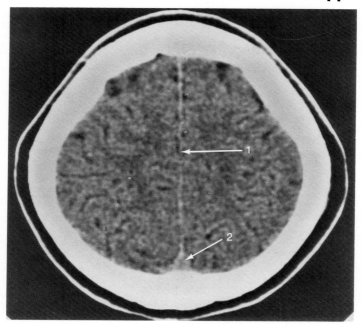

FIG. 10.
1, falx
2, superior sagittal sinus

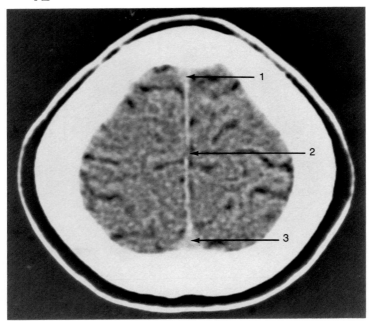

FIG. 11.
1, superior sagittal sinus
2, falx
3, superior sagittal sinus

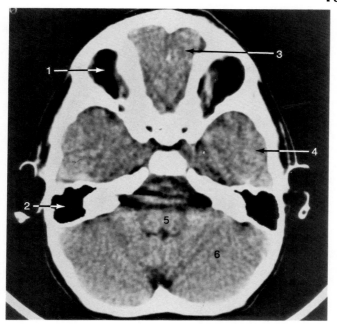

FIG. 12.
1, orbit
2, mastoid air cells
3, frontal lobe
4, temporal lobe
5, medulla
6, cerebellar hemisphere

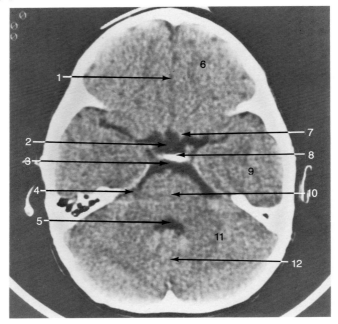

FIG. 13.
1, interhemispheric fissure
2, suprasellar cistern
3, prepontine cistern
4, cerebellopontine angle cistern
5, 4th ventricle
6, frontal lobe
7, optic nerve
8, dorsum sellae
9, temporal lobe
10, pons
11, cerebellar hemisphere
12, cerebellar vermis

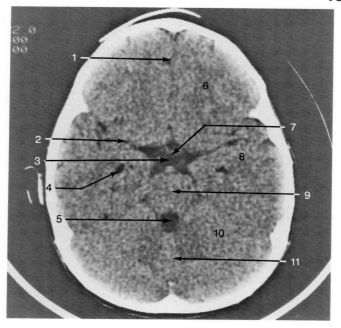

FIG. 14.
1, interhemispheric fissure
2, Sylvian cistern
3, suprasellar cistern
4, temporal horn
5, 4th ventricle
6, frontal lobe
7, optic chiasm
8, temporal lobe
9, pons
10, cerebellar hemisphere
11, cerebellar vermis

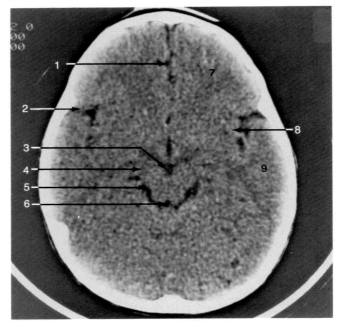

FIG. 15.
1, interhemispheric fissure
2, Sylvian fissure
3, interpeduncular cistern
4, crural cistern
5, ambient cistern
6, cerebral aqueduct
7, frontal lobe
8, insula
9, temporal lobe

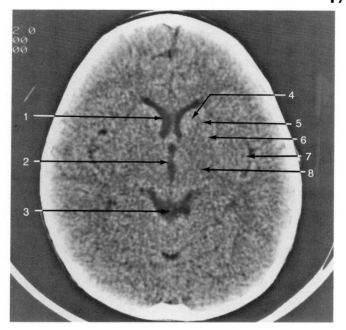

FIG. 16.
1, frontal horn
2, 3rd ventricle
3, quadrigeminal cistern
4, head of caudate nucleus
5, anterior limb of internal capsule
6, lentiform nucleus
7, insula
8, posterior limb of internal capsule

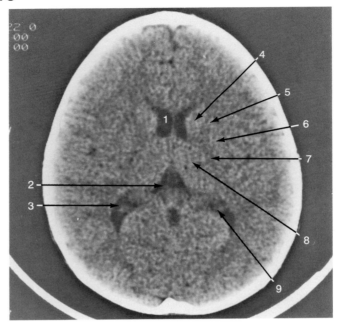

FIG. 17.
1, frontal horn
2, cistern of velum interposium
3, trigone
4, head of caudate nucleus
5, anterior limb of internal capsule
6, lentiform nucleus
7, posterior limb of internal capsule
8, thalamus
9, choroid plexus

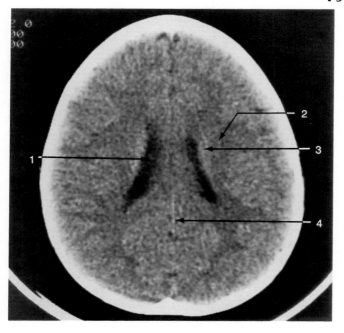

FIG. 18.
1, body of lateral ventricle
2, corona radiata
3, body of caudate nucleus
4, falx

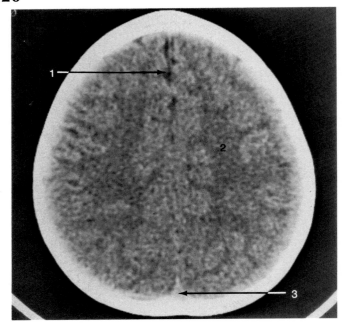

FIG. 19.
1, interhemispheric fissure
2, centrum semiovale
3, superior sagittal sinus

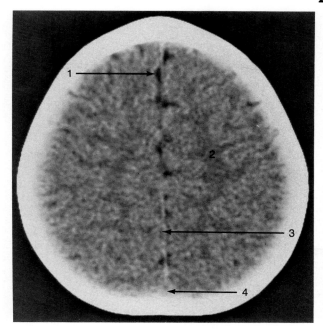

FIG. 20.
1, interhemispheric fissure
2, centrum semiovale
3, falx
4, superior sagittal sinus

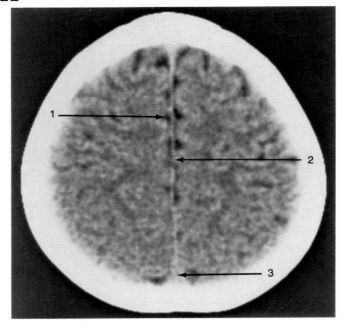

FIG. 21.
1, interhemispheric fissure
2, falx
3, superior sagittal sinus

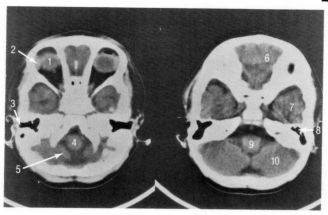

FIG. 22.
   1, ocular bulb
   2, lacrimal gland
   3, external auditory canal
   4, medulla
   5, cerebellar tonsil
   6, frontal lobe
   7, temporal lobe
   8, mastoid air cells
   9, medulla
10, cerebellar hemisphere

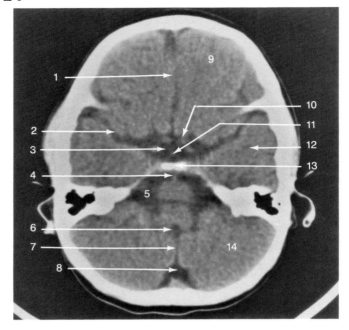

FIG. 23.
1, interhemispheric fissure
2, Sylvian cistern
3, suprasellar cistern
4, prepontine cistern
5, cerebellopontine angle cistern
6, 4th ventricle
7, vallecula
8, cisterna magna
9, frontal lobe
10, optic nerve
11, infundibulum
12, temporal lobe
13, dorsum sellae
14, cerebellar hemisphere

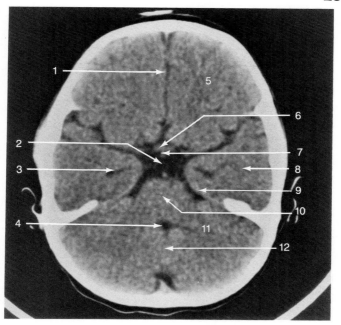

FIG. 24.
1, interhemispheric fissure
2, suprasellar cistern
3, temporal horn
4, 4th ventricle
5, frontal lobe
6, optic chiasm
7, infundibulum
8, temporal lobe
9, tentorium
10, pons
11, cerebellar hemisphere
12, cerebellar vermis

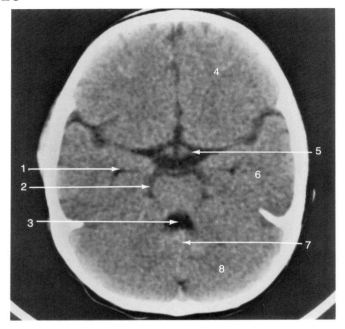

FIG. 25.
1, temporal horn
2, crural cistern
3, 4th ventricle
4, frontal lobe
5, optic tract
6, temporal lobe
7, cerebellar vermis
8, cerebellar hemisphere

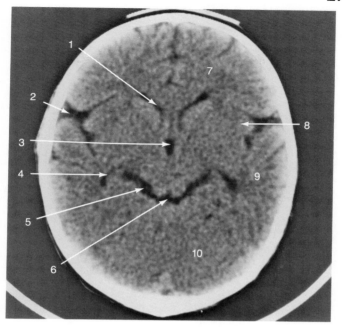

FIG. 26.
1, frontal horn
2, Sylvian fissure
3, 3rd ventricle
4, temporal horn
5, ambient cistern
6, quadrigeminal cistern
7, frontal lobe
8, insula
9, temporal lobe
10, cerebellar hemisphere

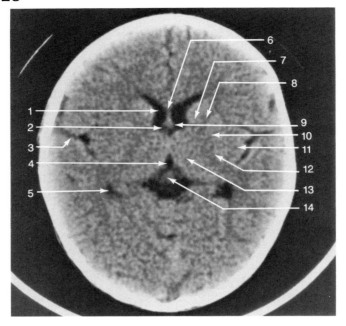

FIG. 27.
1, frontal horn
2, foramen of Monro
3, Sylvian fissure
4, 3rd ventricle
5, temporal horn
6, corpus callosum
7, head of caudate nucleus
8, anterior limb of internal capsule
9, fornix
10, lentiform nucleus
11, insula
12, posterior limb of internal capsule
13, thalamus
14, pineal gland

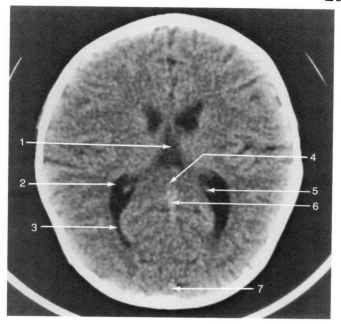

FIG. 28.
1, cavum vergae
2, trigone
3, occipital horn
4, corpus callosum
5, choroid plexus
6, inferior sagittal sinus
7, superior sagittal sinus

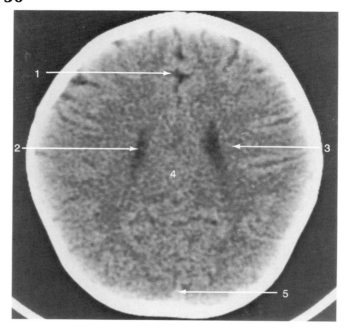

FIG. 29.
1, interhemispheric fissure
2, body of lateral ventricle
3, corona radiata
4, body of corpus callosum
5, superior sagittal sinus

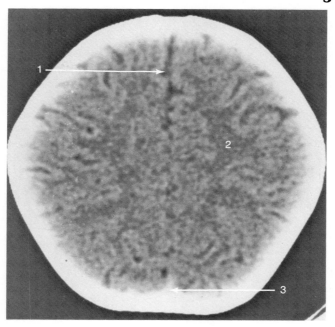

FIG. 30.
1, interhemispheric fissure
2, centrum semiovale
3, superior sagittal sinus

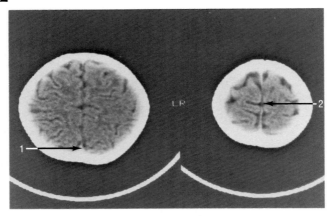

FIG. 31.
1, superior sagittal sinus
2, falx

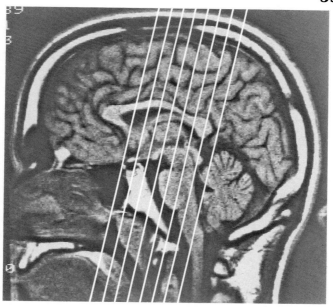

FIG. 32.
Coronal

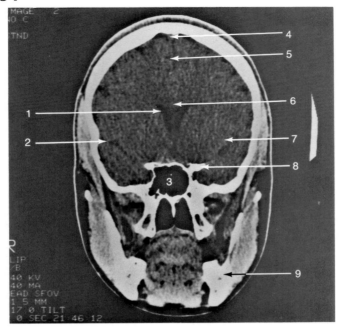

FIG. 33.
1, lateral ventricle (frontal horn)
2, Sylvian fissure
3, sphenoid sinus
4, superior sagittal sinus
5, falx
6, corpus callosum
7, insula
8, anterior clinoid process
9, mandible

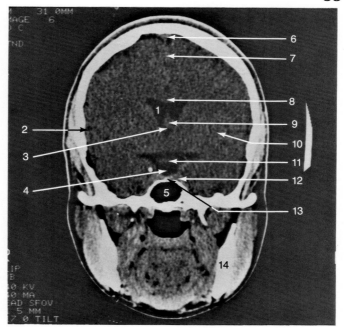

FIG. 34.
1, lateral ventricle
2, Sylvian fissure
3, 3rd ventricle
4, suprasellar cistern
5, sphenoid sinus
6, superior sagittal sinus
7, falx
8, corpus callosum
9, fornix
10, insula
11, optic chiasm
12, cavernous sinus
13, pituitary gland
14, mandible

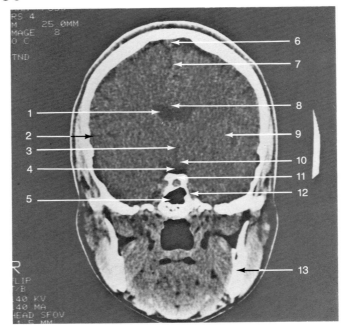

FIG. 35.
1, lateral ventricle
2, Sylvian fissure
3, 3rd ventricle
4, suprasellar cistern
5, sphenoid sinus
6, superior sagittal sinus
7, falx
8, corpus callosum
9, insula
10, hypothalamus
11, dorsum sellae
12, cavernous sinus
13, mandible

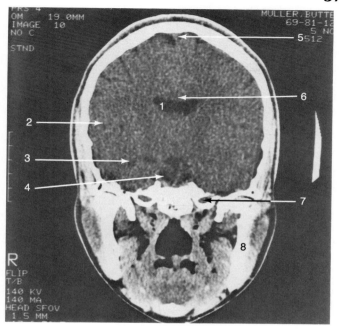

FIG. 36.
1, lateral ventricle
2, Sylvian fissure
3, lateral ventricle (temporal horn)
4, prepontine cistern
5, superior sagittal sinus
6, corpus callosum
7, carotid canal
8, mandible

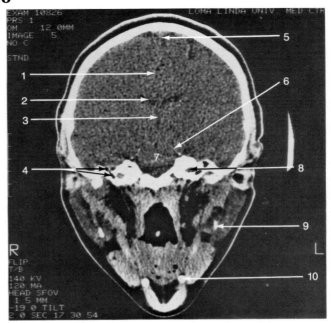

FIG. 37.

1, interhemispheric fissure
2, lateral ventricle
3, 3rd ventricle
4, middle ear
5, superior sagittal sinus
6, tentorium
7, pons
8, carotid canal
9, mandible
10, hyoid bone

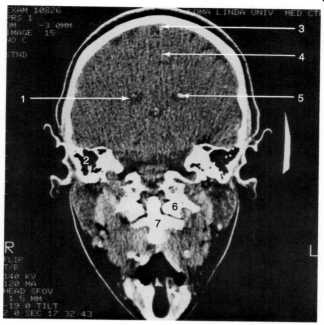

FIG. 38.
1, lateral ventricle
2, mastoid air cells
3, superior sagittal sinus
4, falx
5, choroid plexus
6, C_1
7, C_2

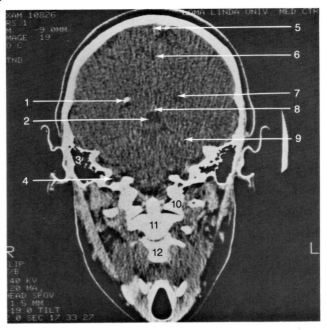

FIG. 39.
1, choroid plexus
2, quadrigeminal cistern
3, mastoid air cells
4, jugular canal
5, superior sagittal sinus
6, falx
7, lateral ventricle
8, vein of Galen
9, tentorium
10, C_1
11, C_2
12, C_3

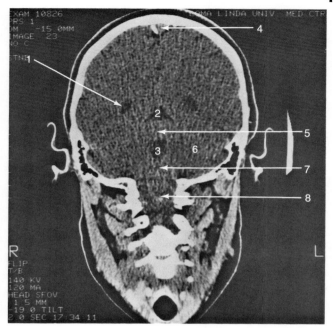

FIG. 40.
1, lateral ventricle
2, superior cerebellar cistern
3, 4th ventricle
4, superior sagittal sinus
5, cerebellar vermis
6, cerebellar hemisphere
7, medulla
8, cervical spinal cord

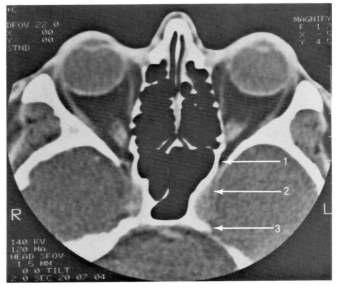

FIG. 41.
1, superior orbital fissure
2, first division of trigeminal nerve
3, gasserian ganglion

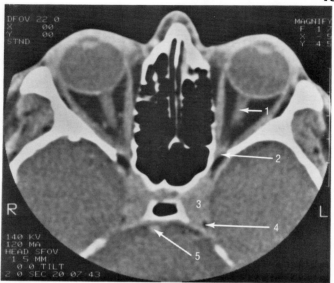

FIG. 42.
1, optic nerve
2, superior orbital fissure
3, cavernous sinus
4, Meckel's cavity
5, basilar artery

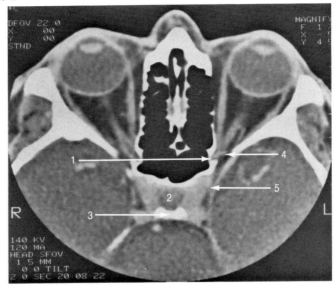

FIG. 43.
1, optic canal
2, pituitary gland
3, dorsum sellae
4, superior orbital fissure
5, oculomotor nerve

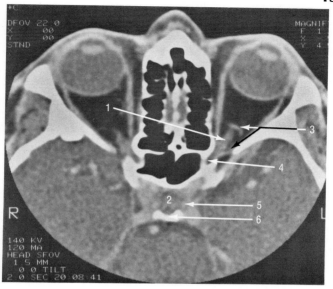

FIG. 44.
1, optic nerve
2, pituitary gland
3, ophthalmic artery
4, optic canal
5, cavernous sinus
6, dorsum sellae

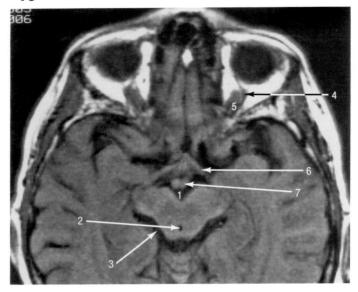

FIG. 45. MRI (T1 Weighted Axial Image)
1, interpeduncular cistern
2, cerebral aqueduct
3, ambient cistern
4, ophthalmic artery
5, optic nerve
6, optic tract
7, mamillary body

Temporal Bone, Skull Base, and Sella _____

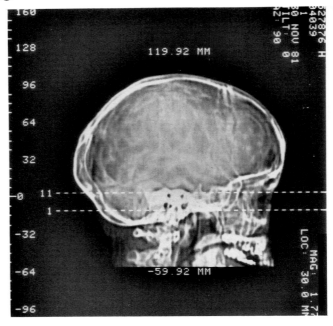

FIG. 1.

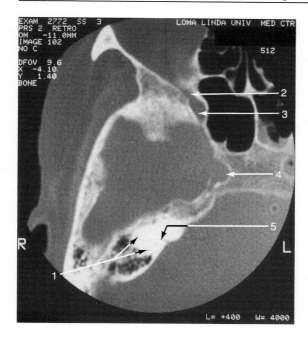

FIG. 2.
1, superior semicircular canal
2, superior orbital fissure
3, pterygopalatine fossa
4, carotid canal
5, petromastoid canal

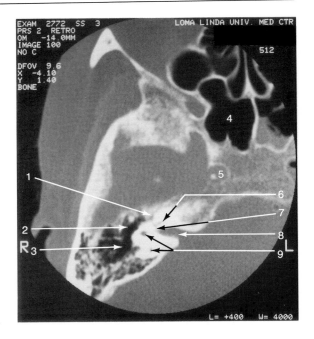

FIG. 3.
1, geniculate ganglion
2, epitympanum
3, antrum
4, sphenoid sinus
5, carotid canal
6, cochlea (basal turn)
7, facial canal
8, internal auditory canal
9, superior semicircular canal

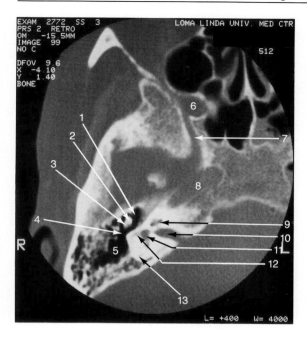

FIG. 4.
1, epitympanum
2, malleus (head)
3, incus (body)
4, aditus ad antrum
5, antrum
6, pterygopalatine fossa
7, foramen rotundum
8, carotid canal
9, cochlea
10, internal auditory canal
11, vestibule
12, lateral semicircular canal
13, posterior semicircular canal

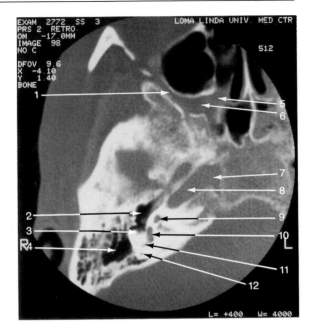

FIG. 5.
1, inferior orbital fissure
2, epitympanum
3, facial canal
4, antrum
5, sphenopalatine fossa
6, pterygopalatine fossa
7, foramen lacerum
8, carotid canal
9, cochlea
10, vestibule
11, lateral semicircular canal
12, posterior semicircular canal

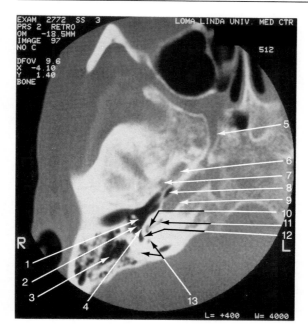

FIG. 6.
   1, malleus (handle)
   2, incus (long process)
   3, antrum
   4, stapes
   5, vidian (pterygoid) canal
   6, foramen ovale
   7, foramen spinosum
   8, auditory tube
   9, carotid canal
   10, vestibule
   11, cochlea (basal turn)
   12, tympanic sinus
   13, posterior semicircular canal

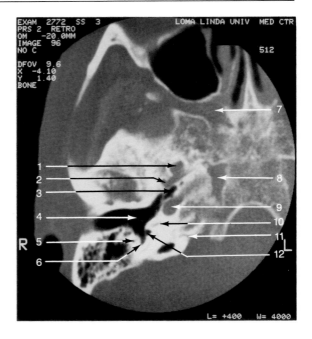

FIG. 7.
1, foramen ovale
2, foramen spinosum
3, auditory tube
4, malleus (handle)
5, facial canal
6, tympanic sinus
7, pterygopalatine fossa
8, foramen lacerum
9, carotid canal
10, cochlea (basal turn)
11, cochlear aqueduct
12, round window

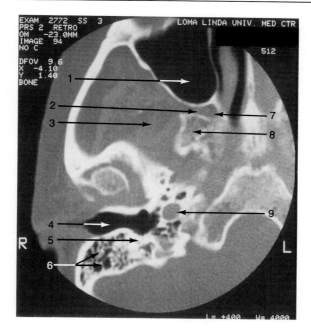

FIG. 8
1, maxillary sinus
2, pterygomaxillary fissure
3, infratemporal fossa
4, external auditory canal
5, facial canal
6, mastoid air cells
7, pterygopalatine fossa
8, pterygoid process
9, carotid canal

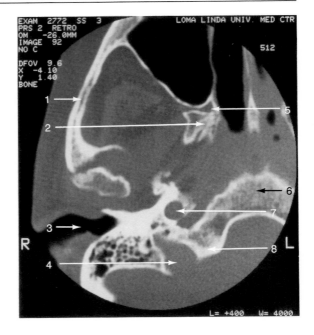

FIG. 9.
1, zygomatic arch
2, pterygoid process
3, external auditory canal
4, jugular foramen
5, pterygopalatine foramen
6, clivus
7, carotid canal
8, jugular tubercle

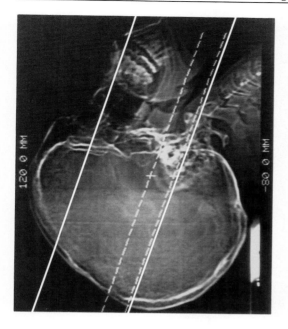

FIG. 10.
Coronal

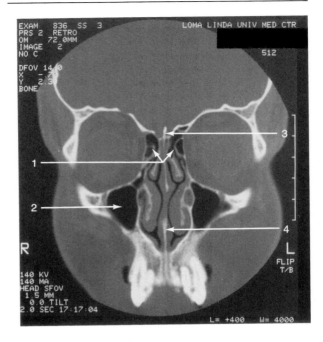

FIG. 11.
1, ethmoid air cells
2, maxillary sinus
3, crista galli
4, nasal septum

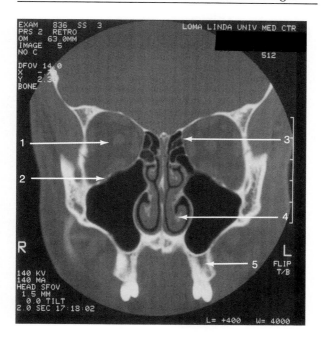

FIG. 12.
1, orbit
2, infraorbital foramen
3, lamina papyracea
4, inferior nasal turbinate
5, maxilla (alveolar process)

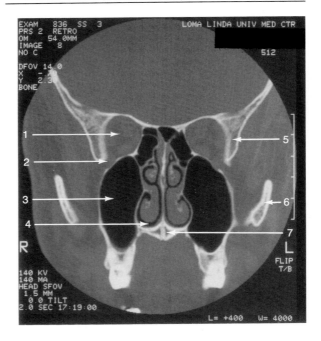

FIG. 13.
1, orbit
2, inferior orbital fissure
3, maxillary sinus
4, nasal cavity
5, sphenoid bone (greater wing)
6, zygomatic arch
7, hard palate

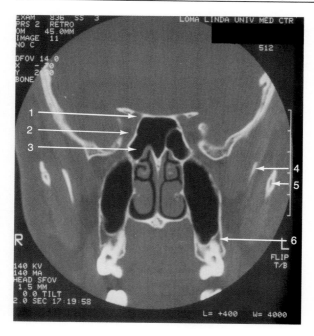

FIG. 14.
1, optic canal
2, superior orbital fissure
3, sphenoid sinus
4, mandible
5, zygomatic arch
6, maxilla (alveolar process)

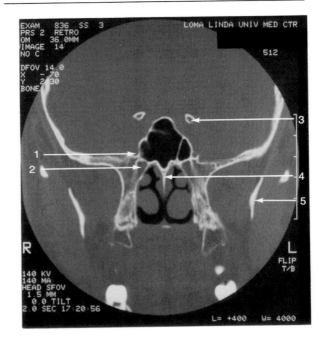

FIG. 15.
1, foramen rotundum
2, pterygopalatine fossa
3, anterior clinoid process
4, vomer
5, mandible

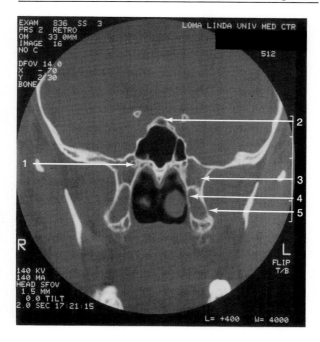

FIG. 16.
1, vidian (pterygoid) canal
2, tuberculum sellae
3, sphenoid bone (pterygoid process)
4, medial pterygoid plate
5, lateral pterygoid plate

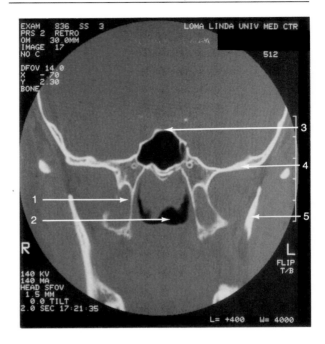

FIG. 17.
1, pterygoid fossa
2, nasopharynx
3, floor of sella turcica
4, floor of middle fossa
5, mandible

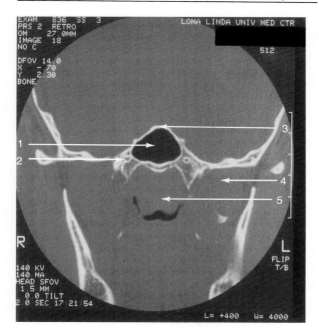

FIG. 18.

1, sphenoid sinus
2, vidian (pterygoid) canal
3, floor of sella turcica
4, infratemporal fossa
5, adenoid tissues

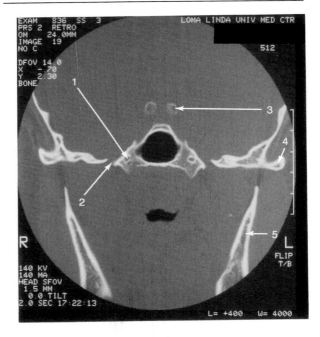

FIG. 19.
1, vidian (pterygoid) canal
2, foramen ovale
3, posterior clinoid process
4, temporal bone (zygomatic process)
5, mandible

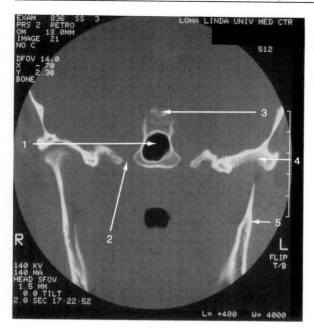

FIG. 20.
1, sphenoid sinus
2, foramen lacerum
3, dorsum sellae
4, temporal bone (glenoid fossa)
5, mandible

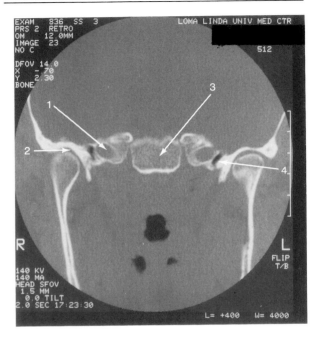

FIG. 21.
1, carotid canal
2, temporomandibular joint
3, clivus
4, auditory tube

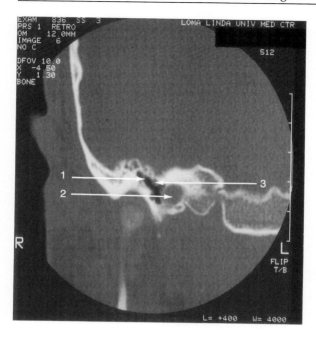

FIG. 22.
1, epitympanum
2, carotid canal
3, geniculate ganglion

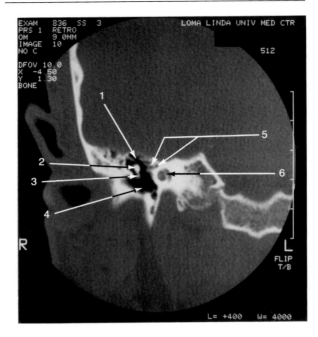

FIG. 23.

1, epitympanum
2, malleus (head)
3, malleus (handle)
4, tympanic membrane
5, facial canal
6, cochlea

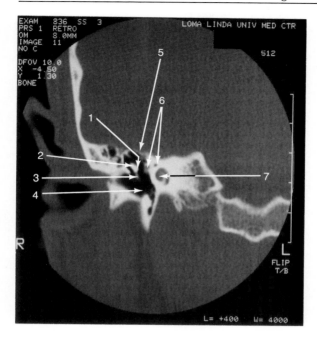

FIG. 24.
1, malleus (head)
2, incus (body)
3, malleus (handle)
4, tympanic membrane
5, tegmen tympani
6, facial canal
7, cochlea

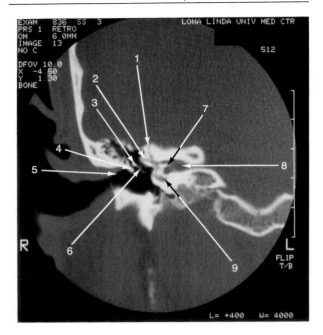

FIG. 25.
1, superior semicircular canal
2, lateral semicircular canal
3, incus (body)
4, scutum
5, external auditory canal
6, incus (long process)
7, falciform crest
8, internal auditory canal
9, cochlea (basal turn)

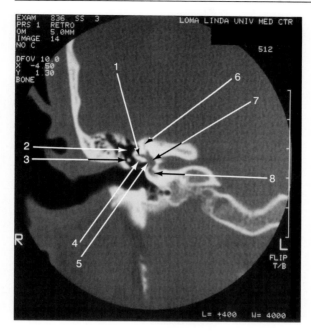

FIG. 26.
1, lateral semicircular canal
2, epitympanum
3, incus (short process)
4, facial nerve
5, oval window
6, superior semicircular canal
7, vestibule
8, cochlea (basal turn)

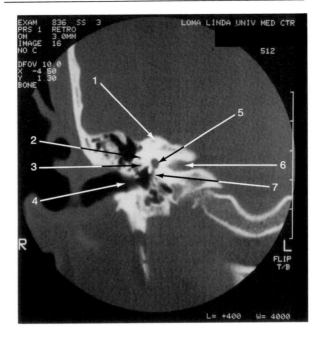

FIG. 27.
1, superior semicircular canal
2, lateral semicircular canal
3, facial canal
4, external auditory canal
5, vestibule
6, internal auditory canal
7, round window

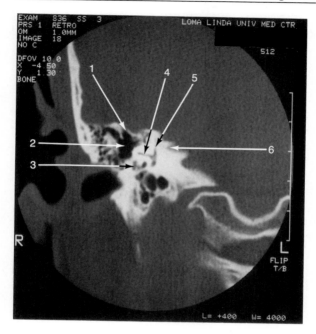

FIG. 28.

1, tegmen antri
2, antrum
3, facial canal
4, lateral semicircular canal
5, superior semicircular canal
6, petromastoid canal

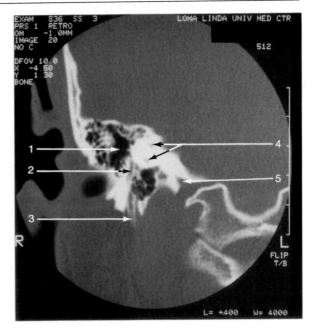

FIG. 29.
1, antrum
2, facial canal
3, styloid process
4, posterior semicircular canal
5, cochlear aqueduct

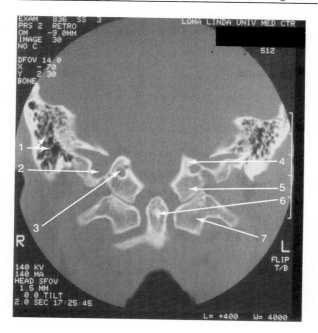

FIG. 30.
1, mastoid air cells
2, jugular foramen
3, hypoglossal canal
4, jugular tubercle
5, occipital condyle
6, odontoid process
7, 1st cervical vertebra (atlas)

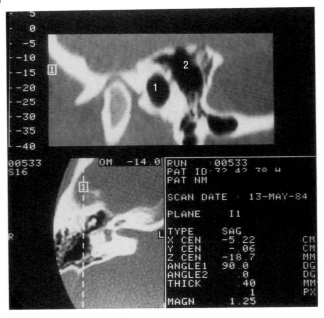

FIG. 31.
1, external auditory canal
2, antrum

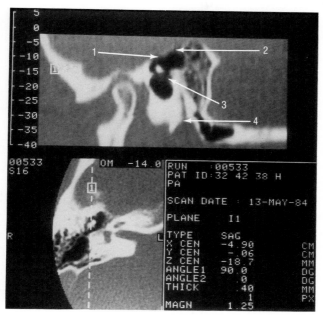

FIG. 32.
1, tegmen tympani
2, tegmen antri
3, attachment of tympanic membrane
4, stylomastoid foramen

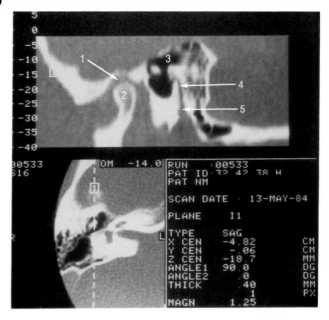

FIG. 33.
1, glenoid fossa
2, mandibular condyle
3, aditus ad antrum
4, facial canal
5, stylomastoid foramen

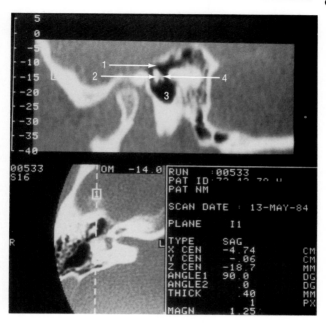

FIG. 34.
1, epitympanum
2, malleus (head)
3, external auditory canal
4, incus (body)

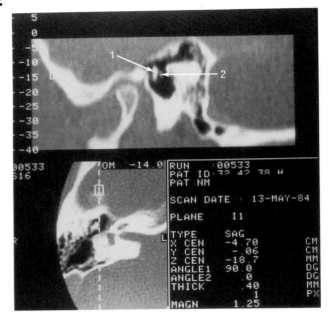

FIG. 35.
1, malleus (head and neck)
2, incus

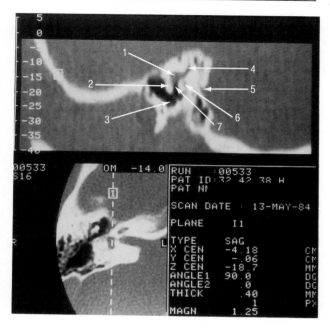

FIG. 36.
1, vestibule
2, promontory
3, tympanic cavity
4, common crus of posterior and superior semicircular
   canal
5, vestibular aqueduct
6, ampulla of posterior semicircular canal
7, round window

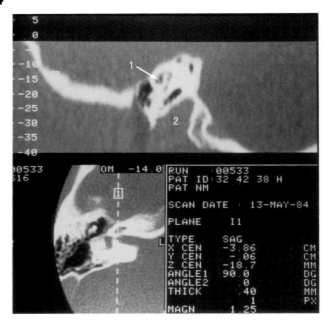

FIG. 37.
1, cochlea
2, jugular fossa

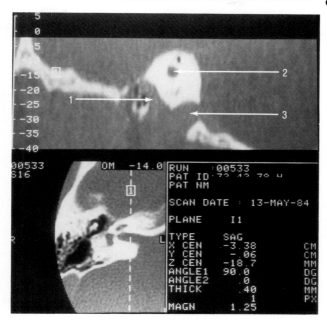

FIG. 38.
1, carotid canal
2, internal auditory canal
3, jugular canal